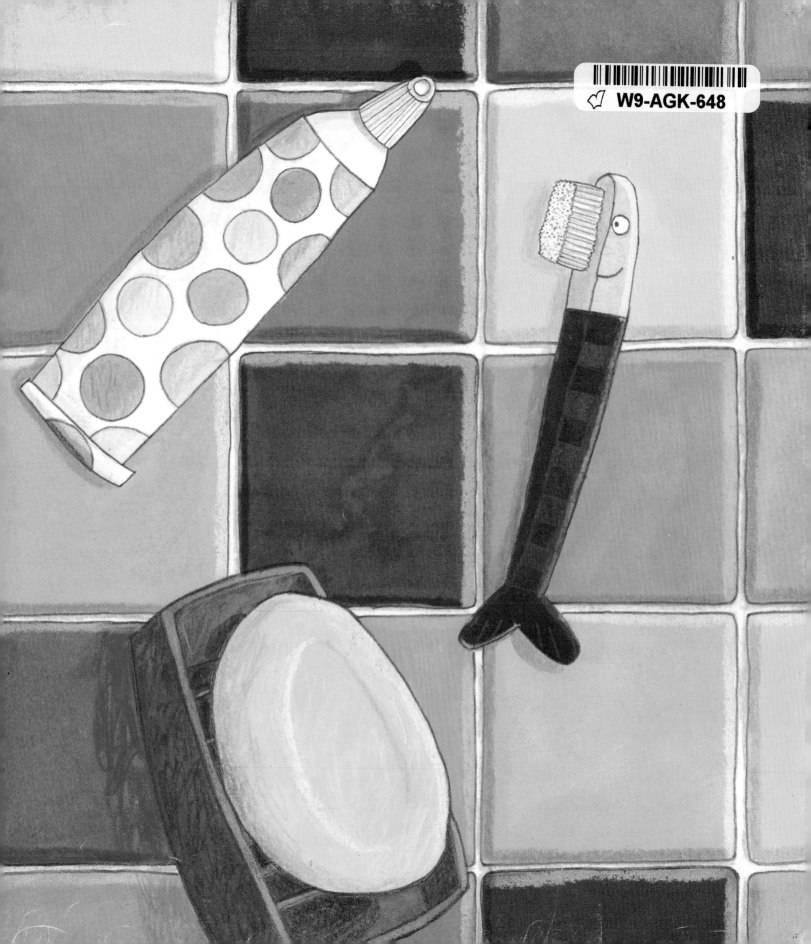

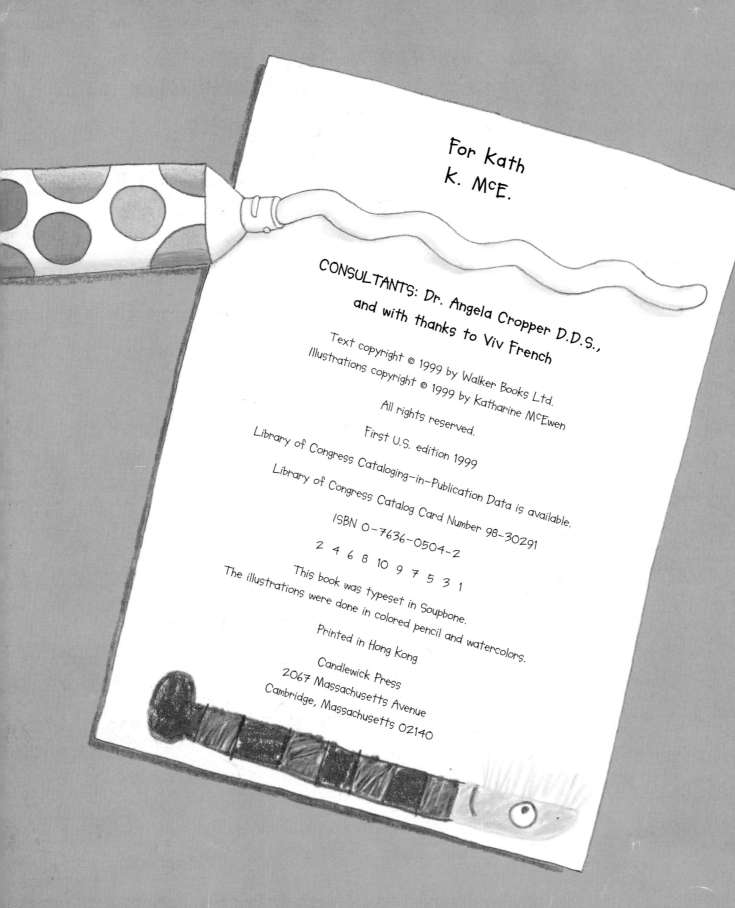

For Kath
K. McE.

CONSULTANTS: Dr. Angela Cropper D.D.S.,
and with thanks to Viv French

Text copyright © 1999 by Walker Books Ltd.
Illustrations copyright © 1999 by Katharine McEwen

First U.S. edition 1999

Library of Congress Cataloging-in-Publication Data is available.

Library of Congress Catalog Card Number 98-30291

ISBN 0-7636-0504-2

2 4 6 8 10 9 7 5 3 1

This book was typeset in Soupbone.
The illustrations were done in colored pencil and watercolors.

Printed in Hong Kong

Candlewick Press
2067 Massachusetts Avenue
Cambridge, Massachusetts 02140

I KNOW WHY I BRUSH MY TEETH

KATE ROWAN

illustrated by

KATHARINE M^cEWEN

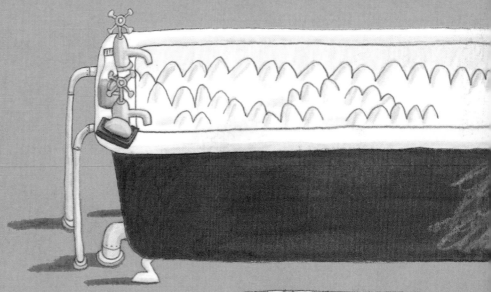

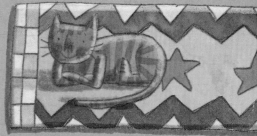

CANDLEWICK PRESS
CAMBRIDGE, MASSACHUSETTS

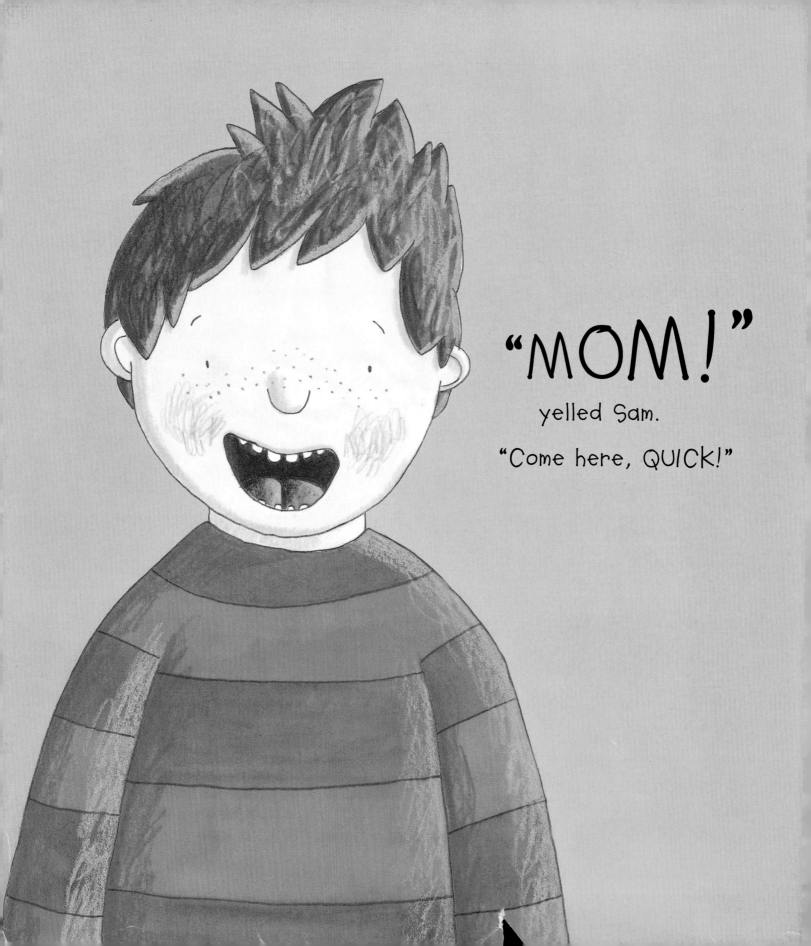

"MOM!"
yelled Sam.

"Come here, QUICK!"

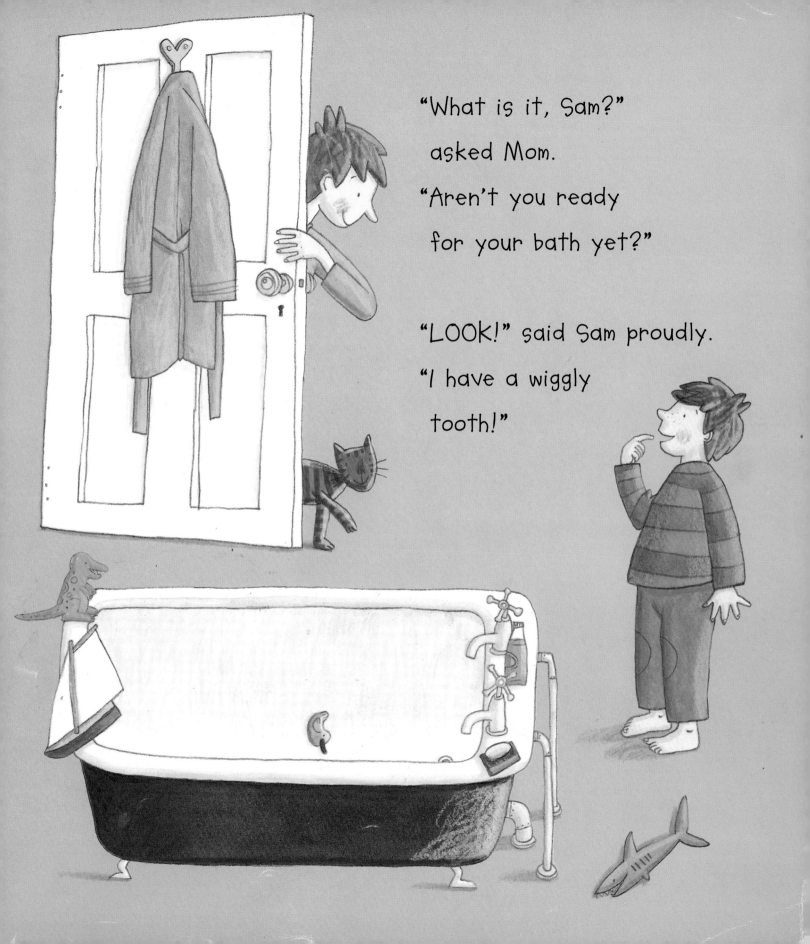

"What is it, Sam?"
asked Mom.
"Aren't you ready
for your bath yet?"

"LOOK!" said Sam proudly.
"I have a wiggly
tooth!"

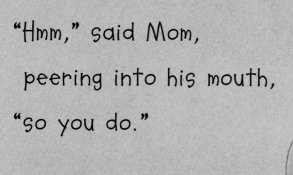

"Hmm," said Mom,
peering into his mouth,
"so you do."

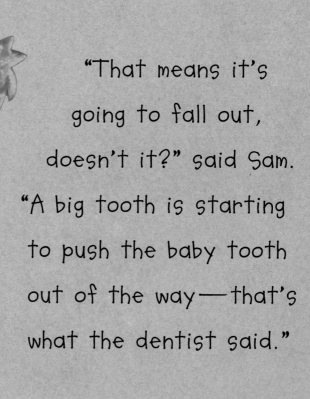

big tooth

baby tooth

gum

JAW BONE

"That means it's
going to fall out,
doesn't it?" said Sam.
"A big tooth is starting
to push the baby tooth
out of the way—that's
what the dentist said."

8

"That's right," Mom said, passing Sam his toothbrush and toothpaste, "but not for a few days yet. So let's give those teeth a really good brushing."

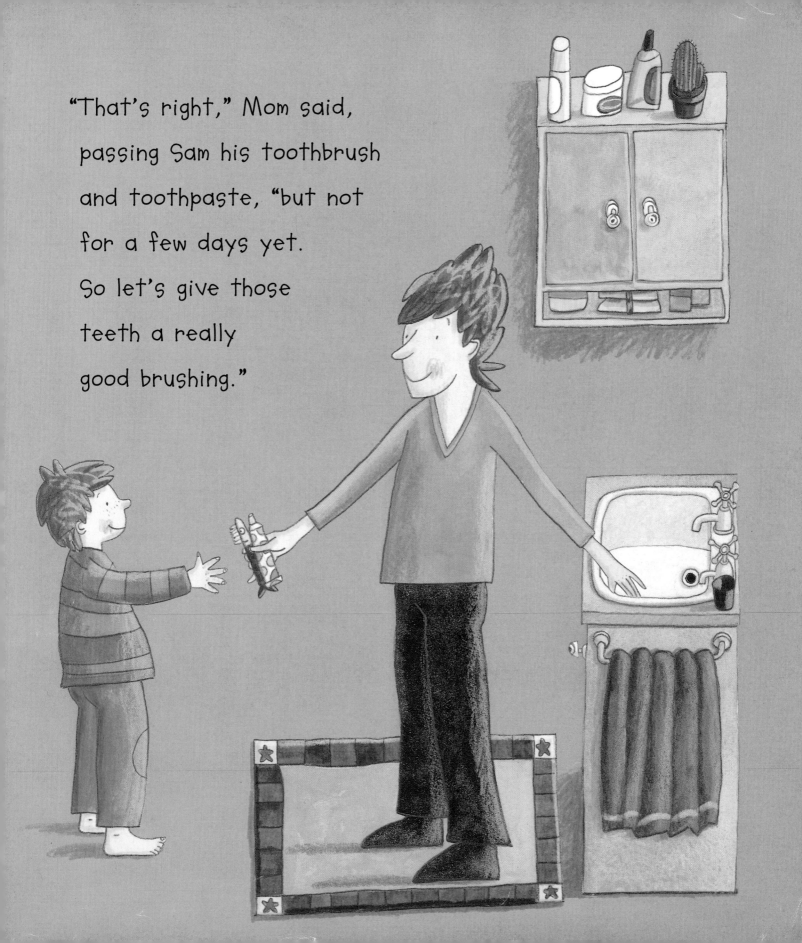

Mom frowned.
"SAM! That's too
much toothpaste!
Remember what else
the dentist said."

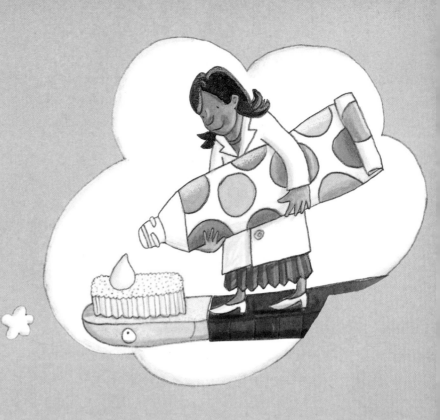

"I know, I know," said Sam.
"Only use a pea-sized drop
of toothpaste, 'cause it has
floor stuff in it, and
I only need a little
of the floor stuff."

"You mean **fluoride**," said Mom.

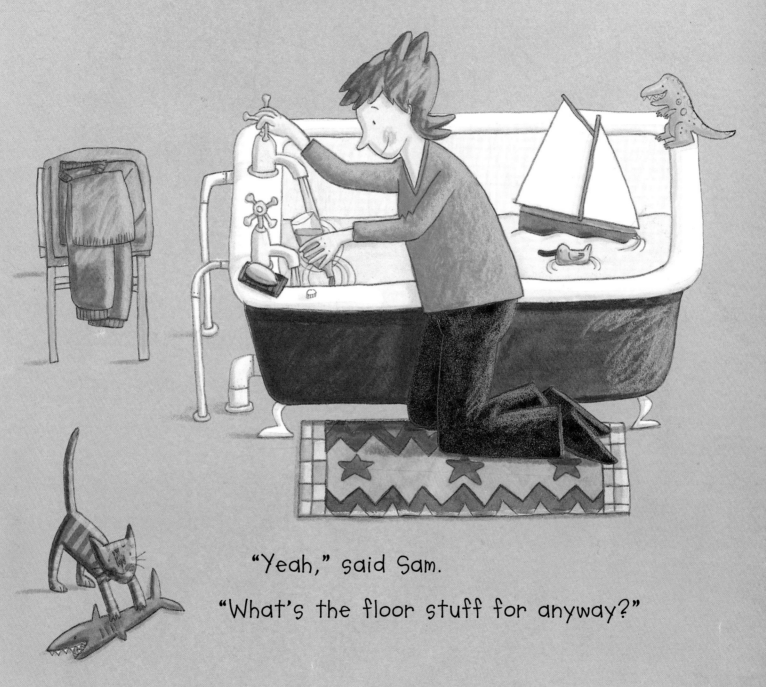

"Yeah," said Sam.

"What's the floor stuff for anyway?"

"It helps to keep your teeth strong," explained Mom.

"I have strong teeth," Sam said. "AND I don't have any holes in them. Jody in my class has holes. Her mom says it's 'cause she eats too much candy."

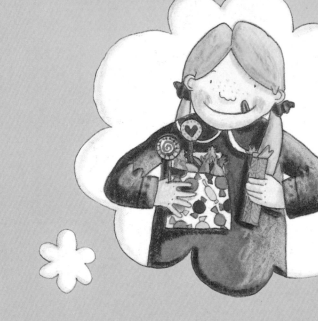

"I suppose it is," said Mom. "Poor Jody. It's not just candy that gives you holes, though. Sugary drinks and snacks between meals aren't good for your teeth either, especially if you don't clean them often enough. That's why you should brush your teeth correctly at least twice a day."

"I know what the right way is," Sam said. "The dentist showed me. Open wide and scrub back and forth along the tops and insides. Then put your teeth together and go around and around on the outsides. Look, I'll show you."

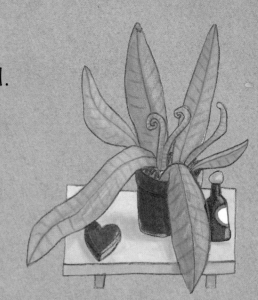

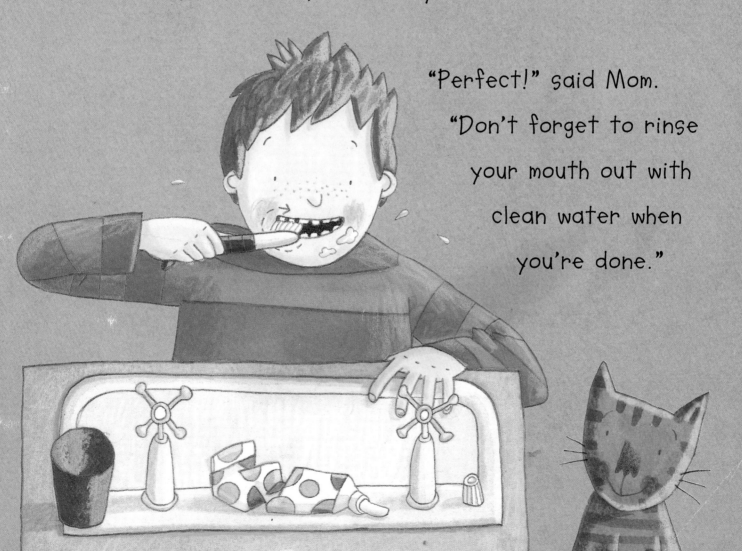

"Perfect!" said Mom. "Don't forget to rinse your mouth out with clean water when you're done."

Sam peered at his
teeth in the mirror.
"Why does brushing
stop the holes?"

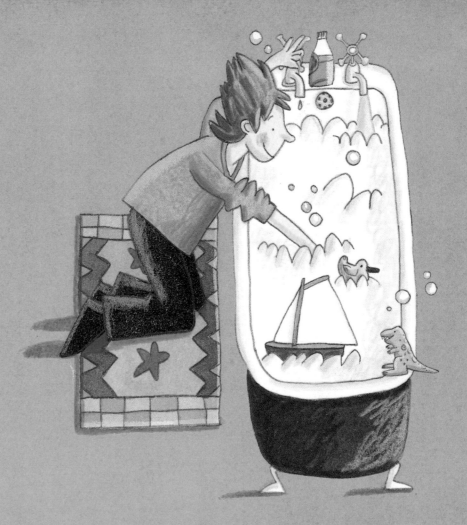

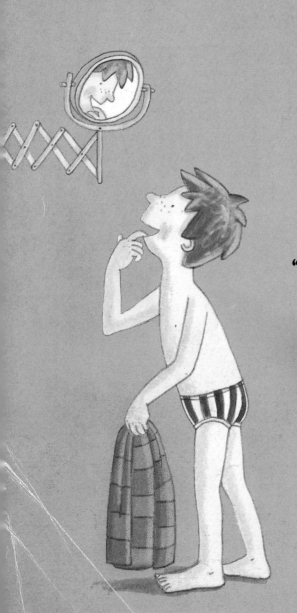

"Because little bits
of food stick to your teeth
when you eat," said Mom.
"If you don't brush them away,
germs called **bacteria** get to work
on them, and form gooey stuff
that builds up on your teeth."

"The gooey stuff's called **plaque**," explained Mom, "and the **bacteria** in the **plaque** feed on the sugar in the food bits. This makes a very strong liquid called **acid**, which eats into the outside of your teeth and makes holes in them."

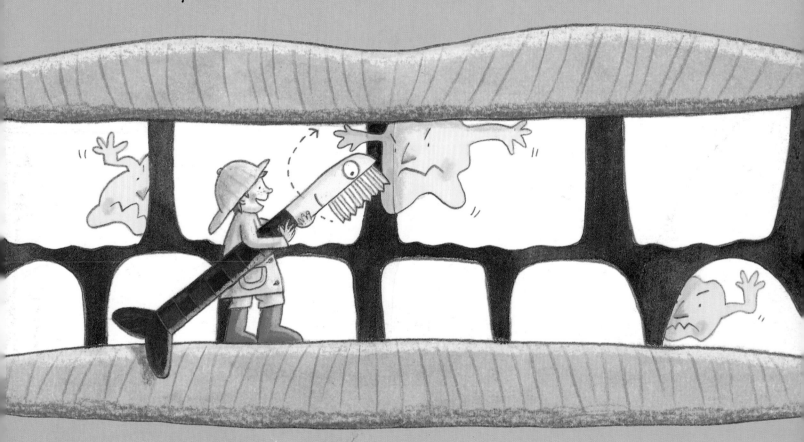

"Oh," said Sam, as he climbed into the bathtub. "Do teeth have an outside and an inside?"

"Yes, they do," said Mom. "The shiny white stuff on the outside is called **enamel**, and it's really hard, like armor. In fact, **enamel** is the hardest thing in your whole body!"

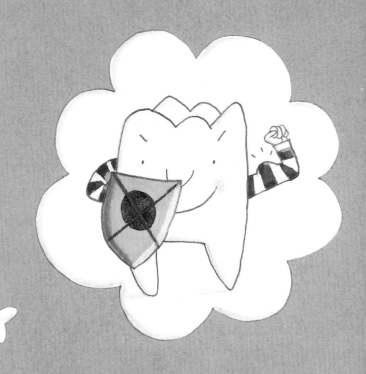

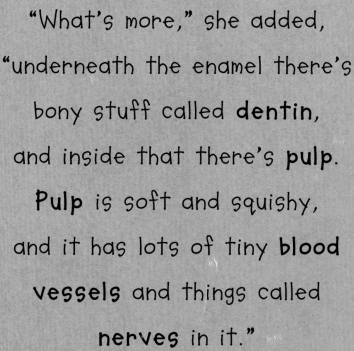

"What's more," she added, "underneath the enamel there's bony stuff called **dentin**, and inside that there's **pulp**. **Pulp** is soft and squishy, and it has lots of tiny **blood vessels** and things called **nerves** in it."

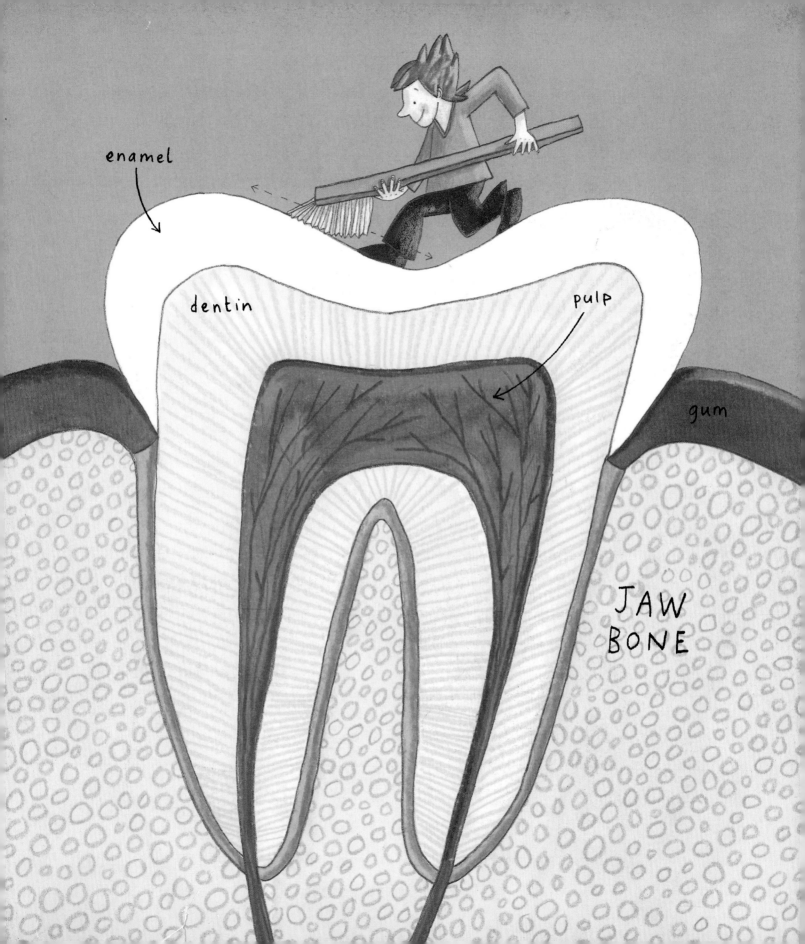

"I know about **nerves**," Sam said. "When I touch something, they tell me if it's hot or cold."

"That's one of the things they do," said Mom. "**Nerves** tell you when something's hurting you, too—like that time I had a hole in one of my teeth and I had a toothache."

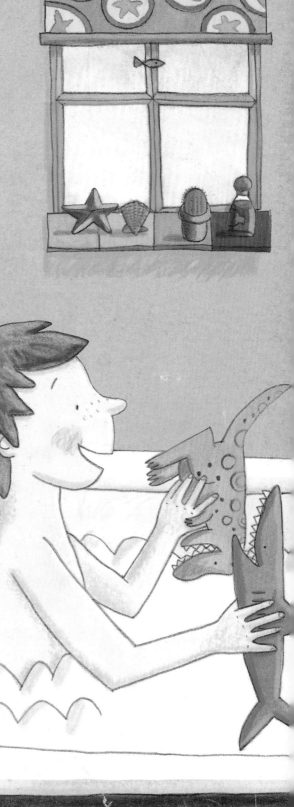

Sam made a face. "Yuck! I hope I never have a toothache."

Mom smiled. "I hope you don't either, but that's why it's so important to take care of your teeth. You'll only grow one set of big teeth, and they'll have to last you the rest of your life."

"Will ALL my baby teeth fall out now?" asked Sam.

"They will," said Mom, "but not all at once. You have twenty baby teeth altogether, and they'll come out one at a time over the next few years."

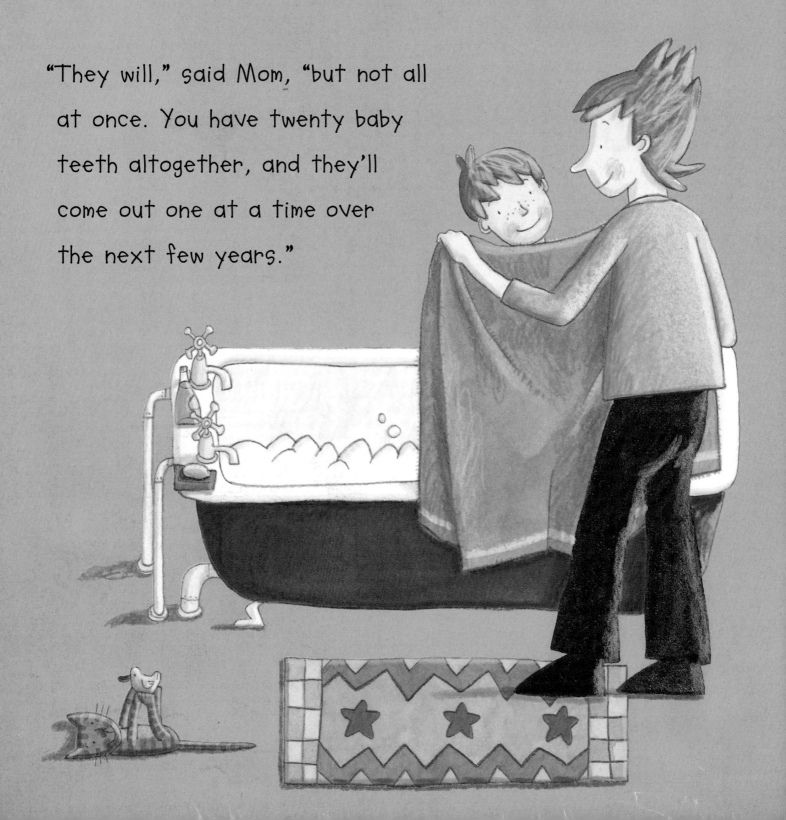

"I know why they're called baby teeth," Sam said. "It's because they started growing when I was a baby. But I'm not a baby anymore, am I? That's why my big teeth are coming in!"

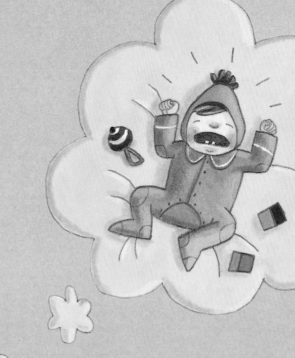

"That's right," said Mom. "You'll get thirty-two big teeth, and you'll have most of them by the time you're thirteen. But you won't get the very last ones, your **wisdom teeth**, until you're a little older."

Sam nodded. "When I'm all grown up, you mean."

21

"Why are they called wisdom teeth?" Sam asked.

"Because you'll be older and wiser by the time you get them!" said Mom. "Your other teeth have names, too, you know."

"They do?" asked Sam. "Like what?"

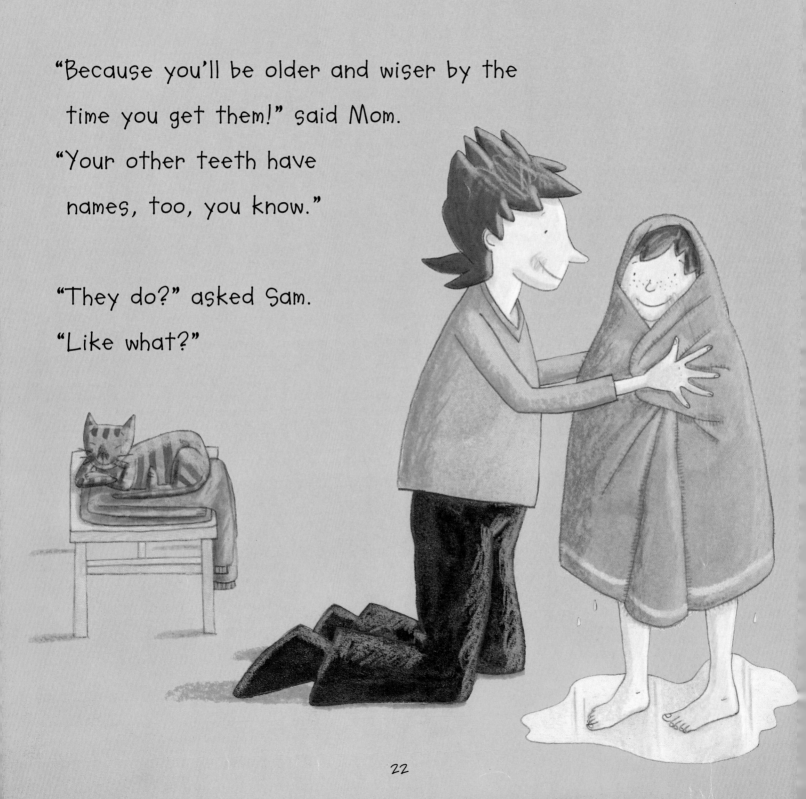

4 incisors
in the middle,
top and bottom

"Well, the teeth at the front are your **incisors**," said Mom. "They work like scissors to cut your food up. And the pointy ones next to them are the **canines**, or dog teeth. They're good for tearing and biting. Then the flat ones at the back are the **molars**. You use those for chewing and grinding up your food."

2 molars on
each side,
top and
bottom

1 canine
on each side,
top and bottom

8 incisors + 8 molars + 4 canines = 20 baby teeth

Sam put on his pajamas.
"Are the dog teeth
called that because
dogs have them, too?"

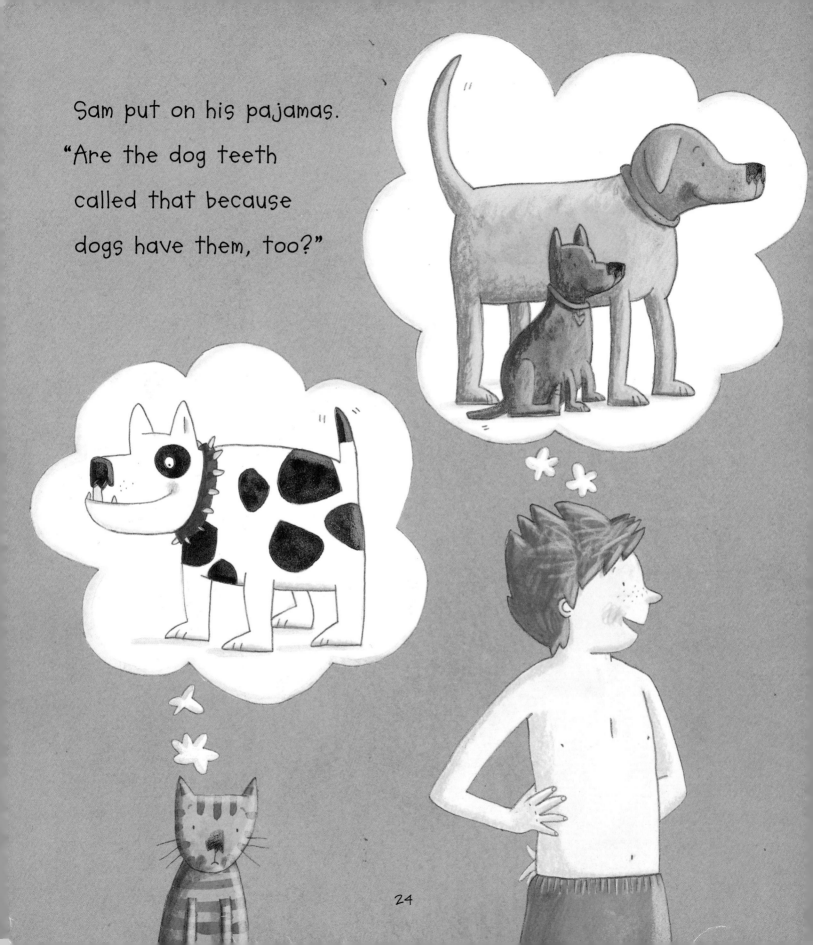

"I think that must be why," Mom said.
"**Canine** is just another
way of saying dog."

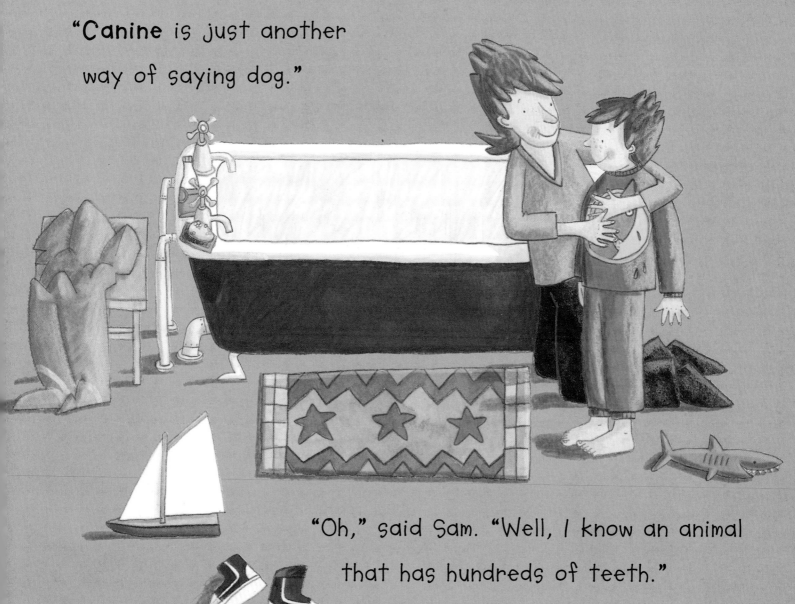

"Oh," said Sam. "Well, I know an animal
that has hundreds of teeth."

Mom laughed.
"You do? What is it?"

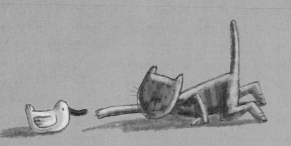

25

"A SHARK!" yelled Sam.

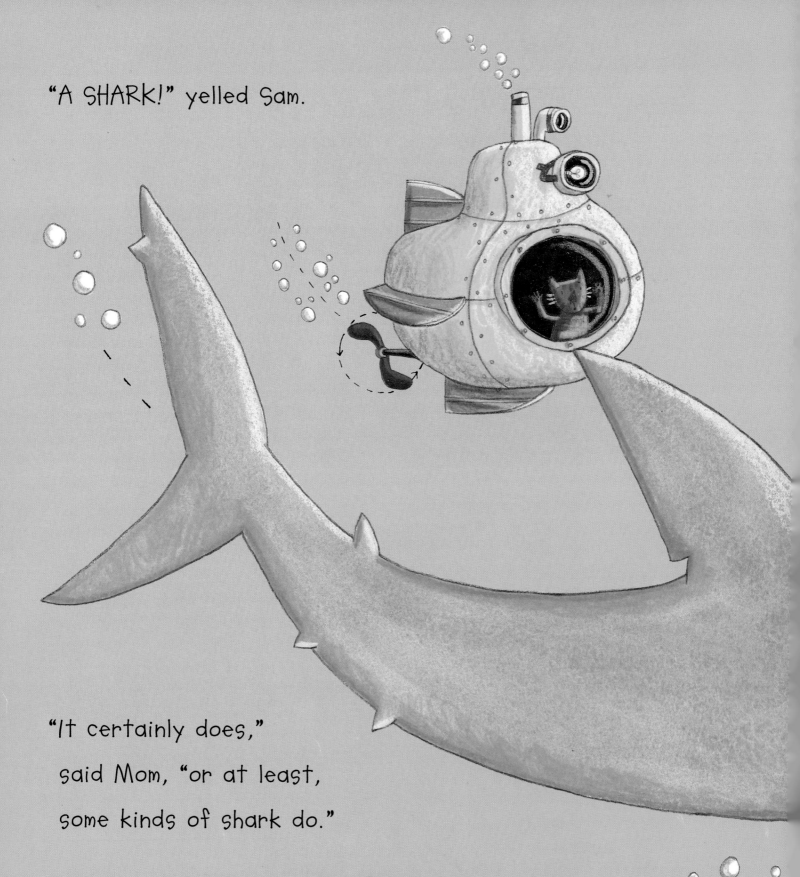

"It certainly does,"
said Mom, "or at least,
some kinds of shark do."

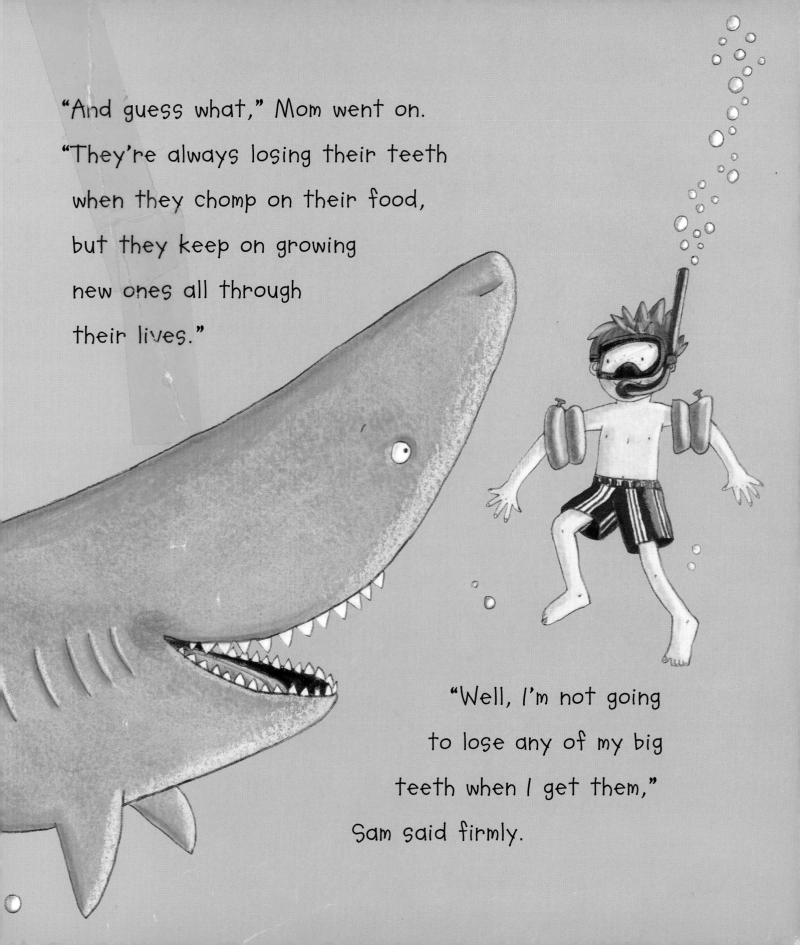

"And guess what," Mom went on.
"They're always losing their teeth
when they chomp on their food,
but they keep on growing
new ones all through
their lives."

"Well, I'm not going
to lose any of my big
teeth when I get them,"
Sam said firmly.

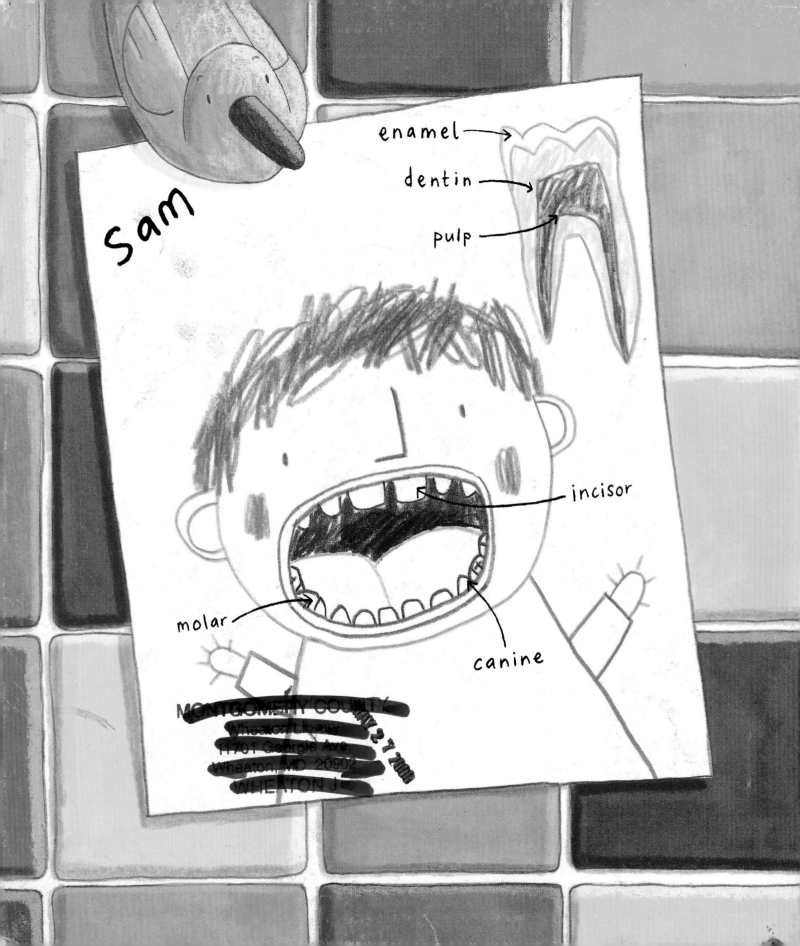